Frequently Asked Questions

all about
chitosan

CAROL SIMONTACCHI, CCN, MS

AVERY PUBLISHING GROUP
Garden City Park • New York

The information contained in this book is based upon the research and personal and professional experiences of the author. It is not intended as a substitute for consulting with your physician or other health care provider. Any attempt to diagnose and treat an illness should be done under the direction of a health care professional.

The publisher does not advocate the use of any particular health care protocol, but believes the information in this book should be available to the public. The publisher and author are not responsible for any adverse effects or consequences resulting from the use of any of the suggestions, preparations, or procedures discussed in this book. Should the reader have any questions concerning the appropriateness of any procedure or preparation mentioned, the author and the publisher strongly suggest consulting a professional health care advisor.

Series cover designer: Eric Macaluso
Cover image courtesy of Barry Axelrod Studios

Avery Publishing Group, Inc.
120 Old Broadway, Garden City Park, NY 11040
1-800-548-5757 or visit us at www.averypublishing.com

ISBN: 0-89529-977-1

Printed in the United States of America

10   9   8   7   6   5   4   3   2   1

Contents

Introduction

If it is difficult for you to imagine life without an occasional order of greasy French fries or a bowl of your favorite ice cream, you may be interested in learning how a natural substance called chitosan (pronounced *ki'-to-san*), a derivative of chitin, absorbs harmful fats before they are deposited in your blood stream (and subsequently on your hips) and escorts them out of your body before they can cause damage.

As Americans, we are all too familiar with diet pills and conventional diets, such as the high-protein diet, the low-calorie diet, the low-fat diet, and the high-carbohydrate diet. We buy exercise equipment, exercise clothes, and exercise videos. We sweat, struggle, and starve. So why do we still gain weight?

The reason for this may be in the food we eat. Studies show that Americans continue to acquire half of their calorie and fat intake from meals outside the home, and that one-third of the individuals who eat out, dine in fast-food restaurants. Pizza is one of the biggest fast-food temptations, while other popular restaurant foods include French fries, hamburgers, and fried chicken. According to one study published in *Nutrition Week*, ". . . the demand for fast, greasy, high-fat foods is growing faster than ever in America."

If we are so concerned with dieting, why has the average amount of fat in the American diet continued to climb since the early 1970s? What are we really saying when we select French fries over a baked potato, or when we choose a hamburger instead of baked fish? Are Americans really as hypocritical as they may seem at first glance?

What we may be saying is that we want to be thin, but we also want to enjoy our food. We want to live a healthy lifestyle, but we don't want to be puritanical about it. In other words, we want to have our cake—low fat of course—and eat it too!

As you read through the chapters of this book, you'll discover that strict adherence to a tasteless, low-fat diet may not always be necessary to lose weight and to improve your overall health. You'll learn how a well-studied natural product from the sea may allow you to cheat occasionally without the accompanying guilt, and how you may lower your risk of certain diseases at the same time.

In *All About Chitosan*, you'll read about the remarkable discovery of this versatile fiber. You'll learn about the incredible benefits that chitosan can bring to the frustrated dieter. You'll also discover that chitosan possesses some additional qualities that can help in the long-term prevention of certain diseases, such as cancer, and certain conditions, such as high cholesterol. You will be supplied with information on the production, dosage, and proper use of chitosan. And you'll also read about the many non-dietary uses of this beneficial fiber.

1.

Chitosan—A Derivative of Chitin

When chitin was originally discovered in the early 1800s, researchers were not looking for a way to remove fat from their bodies. Instead, they discovered an abundant fiber that seemed to have the potential for an incredible variety of applications. It wasn't until the 1980s that researchers began investigating chitosan's use as a dietary supplement. Ivan Furda, PhD, formerly from General Mills, was granted the patent on chitosan's dietary use. The patent is now expired.

Q. Who discovered chitin?

A. In 1811, French researcher Henry Braconnot isolated a unique polysaccharide polymer, or long-chained carbohydrate, called chitin from the cell walls of fungi. Then in 1859, French scientist C. Rougier found chitin in the elytra, or forewings, of the May beetle. Rougier named chitin after the Greek root word meaning *tunic* or *coat of mail*, because he found that chitin comprised about 30 percent of the total cuticle weight of the beetle's forewing. The word chitin was adopted by the English and is in common use today.

Q. What exactly are chitin and chitosan?

A. Some researchers claim that chitin is the second most abundant natural fiber in the world after cellulose, while others insist it is *the* most abundant natural fiber in the world. Either way, chitin is an extremely long chain of sugars and proteins combined to make N-acetyl-D-glucosamine units, or linear copolymers of glucosamine and N-acetylglucosamine.

Chitosan is a chemical derivative of chitin—the combination of sugars and proteins is a little different chemically—and is known as a polycation; a positively charged cation (pronounced *cat-i'-on*) at a biological pH of about six. It is called a hydrocolloid, which means the particles are able to be dispersed in water.

Q. What happens when chitosan is produced from chitin?

A. When chitosan is produced from chitin by the process of deacetylation, acetyl is removed from the molecule, leaving primarily the glucosamine units. These glucosamine molecules are linked together in a long, positively charged chain, giving chitosan some unique properties that make it a valuable fiber for both nutritional and industrial use.

For example, each molecule of chitosan magnetically attaches to fats, also known as fatty acids, which are negatively charged molecules. The combination of the positively charged chitosan and the negatively charged fatty acid is a lump of indigestible material that passes readily out of the body in the process of elimination. Besides being a valuable nutritional supplement, chitosan has many other unique uses that include biomedical applications, paper production, and waste removal.

Q. What is the source of chitosan that we use today?

A. Although chitin was originally sourced from mushrooms and beetles, the most abundant supply of this versatile fiber is in the shells of crustaceans, such as shrimp and crab. Chitin can also be found in krill, clams, oysters, squid, and fungi. Much of the world's current supply of this fiber comes from Japan and Korea. Over 2,000 metric tons of chitosan are produced annually, making it an extremely available source of a natural fiber that can be used in a wide variety of applications.

Q. How is chitosan produced?

A. The process for producing chitosan is relatively simple. First, the crustacean shell is crushed to reduce the size of the particles. Next, the proteins are separated in a chemical bath. Then, the fiber is washed, demineralized using hydrochloric acid, and washed once again. Next, the water is removed, leaving pure chitin. The pure chitin is subjected to the process of deacetylation—the removal of acetyl—and then washed. In the final step, the water is removed, resulting in pure chitosan.

2.

Chitosan's Effect
on Fat

Over time, there has been an incredible diversity of chitosan use in industrial, manufacturing, and agricultural applications. But it was not until American scientist Dr. Ivan Furda began to experiment with chitosan in *in vitro* studies that this unusual fiber's potential was seen in terms of human nutrition. His work clearly demonstrated that chitosan was successful in absorbing free fatty acids in the body. Subsequently, Japanese researchers recognized their abundant source of local crustacean shells and began their own animal and human trials in the early 1980s, resulting in the production of chitosan for dietary purposes.

Q. Why is dietary fat such a problem?

A. The problem with fat is not that we eat too much fat, but that we eat the wrong kinds of fat. Nutritionists are finding that people who consume a typical Western diet are often deficient in essential fatty acids and fat-soluble vitamins, while they have an abundance of fats that cause free-radical damage throughout the body. This free-radical damage can lead to premature aging and a variety of illnesses that could be avoided if people chose, instead, to eat the minimally processed, nutritive oils found in nature.

Q. Where do these harmful free-radical producing fats come from?

A. When highly processed oils are heated to high temperatures, cooled, and then reheated over and over again, they produce free radicals, or carcinogenic agents, that are retained in the prepared food. These carcinogenic agents are introduced into the body when they are eaten and absorbed through the intestinal tract. We might call these harmful fats *biotoxic fats* because they are toxic to life. In other words, they do not promote good health, they hinder it.

Q. How can I protect myself from these harmful fats?

A. One way to help prevent these fats from being absorbed in the body is through the help of chitosan, a unique, biologically active fiber. Researchers have discovered that when chitosan is taken as a supplement, it effectively bonds to dietary fats as they move through the intestinal tract. The chitosan/fat clump is then excreted harmlessly from the body before it is absorbed.

Q. What is fiber?

A. Fiber is generally regarded as the indigestible part of a plant, comprised of different types of materials, such as celluloses, hemicelluloses, pectins, and lignans. Different fibers confer different benefits to the human body, so it is important to consume a wide variety of foods that provide all of the different types of fiber.

Q. How can fiber protect us from the harmful effects of processed fats?

A. As fiber passes through the intestinal tract, it "sweeps" it clean. Fiber also promotes the formation and growth of friendly intestinal bacteria; removes carcinogenic agents from the bowel; removes excess insulin, estrogen, cholesterol, used bile, and other used materials from the body; and helps produce short-chain fatty acids in the intestinal tract. Fiber also stimulates chewing and promotes the flow of saliva; creates a feeling of bulk in the stomach so hunger is satisfied with fewer calories; increases the size of the stool; normalizes intestinal transit time; and slows the digestion and the absorption of nutrients.

Despite all of these beneficial effects, the average American consumes less than 6 g of fiber per day. Nutritionists recommend consuming at least 30 g of fiber per day, along with eight to ten 8-ounce glasses of water.

Q. How does chitosan as a fiber compare to other dietary fibers?

A. Whether or not chitosan is a dietary fiber is still open to discussion, since it does not naturally occur in a form that humans would normally consume. However, chitosan *is* a natural fiber—an indigestible polysaccharide that performs many of the duties that dietary fiber performs, such as decreasing the risk of gastrointestinal disease, certain forms of cancer, heart disease, diabetes, and obesity.

Chitosan is similar to cellulose, a plant fiber, but where chitosan differs from plant fibers is in its magnetic attraction to fat. It doesn't actually sweep the intestinal tract like dietary fiber. Instead, it attracts and attaches to fat and removes it from the body in the fecal material. According to Dr. Furda, chitosan can bind up to fifteen times its weight in lipids or fats in the stomach, far higher than any other type of dietary fiber.

Chitosan does not perform the other essential functions of fiber, so taking chitosan does not substitute for eating vegetables, grains, and fruits. Its task lies simply in removing unwanted fat from the stomach and intestinal tract.

Q. **What happens when I eat fat?**

A. A fat-laden meal, such as a hamburger and fries with a salad that has been tossed with thick dressing and a piece of pie with ice cream on top for dessert—and of course, a cup of coffee with heavy cream—is not digested to any significant degree until it reaches the small intestine. Although a high-fat combination such as this passes into the intestine rather slowly, very little digestive activity actually takes place in the stomach.

Once the fat reaches the small intestine, the gall bladder has already reacted to the presence of fat in the stomach and has transferred large amounts of bile into the intestine to begin the work of emulsifying the fat—allowing the fat to pass through the watery medium of the blood—and cleaving the fatty acids into small, readily absorbable units. After the fatty acids have been reduced into single molecules that can be absorbed through the intestinal lining, they are sent into the lymphatic system and then released into the blood stream where some particles are sent to the liver for processing and others are stored for later use.

Technicians who draw blood from a patient a few hours after he or she has consumed a high-fat meal, such as the one described above, note that the patient's blood stream is actually thick with fat! This fat-rich blood moves more slowly through the blood stream before being deposited in the liver or formed into fat cells.

Q. How can chitosan help counteract this process?

A. When a chitosan capsule is taken at the beginning of a high-fat meal, its contents mix with the slowly digesting watery mass in the stomach. Because it is magnetically attracted to fatty molecules, chitosan immediately binds up to fifteen times its own molecular weight in fat, forming clumps of indigestible material in the stomach. These clumps of chitosan and fats are not broken down in the small intestine and digested. Instead, the fibrous blend moves along the intestinal tract and into the colon, where it is passed out of the body in the fecal material. Hence, fat never gets the chance to clog up the arteries by thickening the blood!

Q. Why do excess calories cause me to gain weight?

A. One of the reasons people gain too much weight is that they take in too many calories. In other words, people take in more calories than their bodies can burn off as energy. The body stores these leftover calories as fat to be used at a later time when energy is needed. This is the body's way of saving up for a rainy day. However, for most us, that rainy day never comes and the stores of fat never get converted to energy! We continue to eat too many calories and to burn too few calories, resulting in ongoing problems with weight gain.

Q. What does fat have to do with weight gain?

A. There is no denying that fat makes food taste good and that eating it gives us pleasure and a feeling of fullness, which is why we tend to crave high-fat foods. But fat is loaded with calories, and our waistlines suffer for it! While carbohydrates and proteins yield about 4 calories per gram, fat yields over 9 calories per gram, making fat a calorie-dense substance. While we must not forget that fat is an essential nutrient and that it would be extremely harmful to the body to remove all fat from the diet, we must also remember that most of the fats we consume are not nutritional in nature. These fats have been so highly processed that they are virtually unusable to the body—except to provide it with an abundant supply of calories.

If we ate only highly nutritious fats such as those found in olive oil, avocados, deep-sea fish, and raw nuts and seeds, it is doubtful that we would suffer the consequences associated with eating high-fat foods. Fats that are highly nutritional can only be consumed in moderation before the body feels satisfied, so overconsumption and weight gain are not usually the problem with these foods.

Q. Will chitosan remove calories along with the fat from my diet?

A. Reducing the amount of fat received into your body will reduce your overall calorie intake. But exactly how many calories chitosan will remove from your diet depends on how many fat calories you are consuming. If you eat a typical American diet, you probably consume about 40 percent of your calories in the form of fat. If you average 1,500 calories per day, that is about 600 calories from fat. Most nutritionists agree that keeping fat calories to around 30 percent of your caloric intake is optimal, provided those are good fat calories. For example, fats from vegetables, nuts and seeds, and omega-3 fatty acids from seafood are considered good fats.

Q. What do the studies show about how chitosan works?

A. Researchers in the laboratory at the University of California, Davis, conducted a study in 1989, published in the *Journal of Nutrition*, in which they separated a group of rats into four groups and fed them different types of fiber. One group was fed 5 percent cellulose, the second group was fed 5 percent guar gum, the third group was fed 5 percent konjac manna, and the fourth group received chitosan. The cellulose-fed group served as the control group, since cellulose does not bind bile or dietary fats.

The group that received the chitosan had a significantly lower amount of fat in the intestinal contents than the other three groups, showing that chitosan effectively bound the fats, reducing the amount of free-floating fat in the watery mass.

Another study conducted at the Kyushu University School of Agriculture in 1989, also published in the *Journal of Nutrition*, tested the effect of chitosan on cholesterol and triglycerides found in the lymphatic system of rats. This study tested two factors—how well chitosan worked to bind the fats and whether certain fats were more easily bound than others. Test studies showed that "Chitosan effectively lowered cholesterol absorption more than did guar gum or cellulose, and this effect was more significant when given with safflower or high-oleic safflower oil than with palm oil."

A third study conducted by Vahouny and published in the *American Journal of Clinical Nutrition* compared rats fed either chitosan or a cholesterol-lowering drug known as cholestyramine. The chitosan showed a 51 percent reduction in the absorption of fat. These were better results than those obtained from cholestyramine. Vahouny concluded that "although these agents may act by different mechanisms, the data suggest that chitosan is as effective as cholestyramine in its acute effects on lipid absorption and that, with chronic feeding, both materials cause equivalent adaptive changes..."

Q. Have any studies shown that chitosan may suppress the appetite?

A. When scientists fed chitosan to chicks along with their normal diet of maize and maize starch, they found that the chitosan reduced their overall intake of food by a significant degree. Apparently, the presence of large amounts of fiber in the stomach tends to take the place of real food, causing chicks to be less hungry.

It is not uncommon for humans to experience the same benefit of a high-fiber diet. Fiber takes up a lot of physical room in the stomach, slowing the digestion of food and the release of sugars into the blood stream and increasing the length of time that you feel satisfied. This is a real benefit to dieters!

Q. What results have there been from human studies on chitosan?

A. A study conducted in 1994 at the ARS Medicina in Helsinki, Finland examined the weight reduction efficacy of chitosan. In other words, researchers wanted to know how well chitosan worked to reduce body weight in their subjects. Each patient was given about 1,800 mg of chitosan in capsule form. Their diet was typical of the Western diet, consisting of 40 percent of calories from fat, 40 percent of calories from carbohydrates, and 20 percent of calories from protein.

Of those participants who completed the study, the average weight loss was fifteen pounds in a four-week period for those taking chitosan. The placebo group had only a five-pound weight loss in the same four-week period.

If you have tried a weight-loss program in the past, you'll know that fifteen pounds in a four-week period is an exciting result, especially when you consider that the diets of the study subjects were not Spartan. Even though the amount of calories was low—about 1,000 calories per day—the amount of fat they consumed probably gave the participants a feeling of satiety. After all, fat not only makes the food you eat taste good, it also makes you feel full and satisfied.

3.

The Side Benefits of Chitosan

Even if the benefits of chitosan were reserved solely for weight loss, this substance would still be a very desirable product. But research shows that there are some significant advantages to using chitosan that have little or nothing to do with weight loss. After all, when you remove the free-radical producing, highly processed fats from your diet, your entire body responds positively. And that is just what researchers found when they expanded their research projects to study the effects of chitosan on the entire body.

Q. If my body absorbs less dietary fat because I'm taking chitosan, what happens to my cholesterol levels?

A. This is where the news of chitosan gets even more exciting! Remember the chicks who received chitosan along with their normal diet? Not only did the chicks eat less food, presumably because they were simply not as hungry, but researchers found that their body weight decreased significantly and the ratio of HDL cholesterol (the "good" cholesterol) to total cholesterol was improved as well. Their overall plasma cholesterol dropped too.

Other studies showed the same benefits. When rats were put on a diet that contained large amounts of both cholesterol and chitosan, researchers found that their total cholesterol dropped with no damage to the liver. Often cholesterol-lowering drugs result in liver damage in the form of smaller, yellowish livers, but these rats maintained healthy livers and lower cholesterol with chitosan use.

Similar studies have been done all over the world, showing the same results. Chitosan apparently lowers total cholesterol and improves the ratio between HDL cholesterol and total cholesterol without any accompanying liver damage. Chitosan was also shown to lower the absorption of dietary triglycerides and to help reduce serum triglycerides.

Q. Since a low-fat diet is highly recommended for diabetics, can diabetics benefit by using chitosan?

A. Researchers in Japan studied the effects of chitosan on blood sugar in mice and found that both blood levels of fats and sugars were reduced in their subjects. Two kinds of mice were used in the study—normal mice and non-insulin dependent diabetic mice with low levels of circulating insulin. Chitosan comprised 5 percent of their total food intake, resulting in reduced levels of blood glucose, total cholesterol, and triglycerides in both groups.

When researchers used chitosan in the diets of mice with high levels of blood sugar, they found that blood sugar levels were not affected by the chitosan. They concluded that chitosan can be a useful treatment in lean type, non-insulin dependent diabetes with low levels of insulin.

Q. Is any information available regarding prostaglandin formation and chitosan?

A. Prostaglandins are very powerful hormones that are formed from essential fatty acids and contribute an amazing variety of benefits to the body. Though many prostaglandins are beneficial, others seem to confer harmful effects on the body, such as increasing inflammation, muscle spasms, allergies, and asthma. Prostaglandins in the 1 and 3 (PGE1 and PGE3) series are considered to be beneficial, while prostaglandins in the 2 series (PGE2) are considered to be harmful. Eating a diet that is high in arachidonic acid—which can be found in red meat—results in the conversion of arachidonic acid to the pro-inflammatory prostaglandin 2 hormone.

When researchers injected study animals with inflammatory substances, they found that the animals who received chitosan were less likely to become inflamed because of reduced PGE2 hormones. In animals that did not receive the chitin, PGE2 hormones were elevated about five times higher than the chitosan-fed animals. From this research, it is presumed that chitosan will lower the amount of arachidonic acid in the body, leading to reduced amounts of PGE2, which in turn leads to reduced inflammation wherever it may be produced. Chitosan, therefore, could be a significant benefit to people suffering from chronic inflammation.

Q. **Since low-fat diets have been linked with a lowered risk of cancer, will chitosan help reduce my risk of cancer or other diseases?**

A. It is possible that a low-fat diet can reduce the risk of cancer—especially cancers of the gastrointestinal tract. Some of the markers for the onset of this type of cancer are what doctors call *aberrant crypt foci, cell proliferation, crypt height*, and *crypt circumference*.

The cells of the small intestine turn over more rapidly than the cells in any other part of the body. They are born and then die within a few short hours. The surface of the small intestine is lined with tiny villi, or tiny finger-like projections, that absorb nutrients from the food. Each villus is surrounded by a pouch, or invagination, called a crypt. The role of the crypt is to secrete digestive fluids into the small intestine and to provide a "factory" for the production of new villi cells. The crypts and villi could be called the "peaks and valleys" of the intestinal tract, and are of equal importance in the overall health of the small intestine.

Diseases like celiac disease flatten these peaks and valleys, which disrupts the normal digestive process.

Mice who were fed high molecular weight chitosan along with their normal diet, and then injected with cancer-causing substances experienced the benefits of significant reductions in the number of aberrant crypt foci, cell proliferation, crypt height, and crypt circumference in the small intestine, thus reducing their risk of subsequent cancer formation.

Q. Can chitosan be used to help prevent other types of cancers?

A. This research is ongoing, but so far, no clinical trials have been recorded regarding chitosan and other types of cancer. However, because highly processed fats have been shown to increase the risk of several other types of cancer, such as breast cancer, prostate cancer, stomach cancer, and liver cancer, it is likely that the risk of developing other forms of cancer would be reduced on a diet that includes chitosan, as well. Furthermore, as I mentioned in Chapter 2, different types of fibers confer different types of benefits to the body, so it would be prudent to include a wide variety of high-fiber foods in your diet. When seeking to prevent cancer, it is best to use all the tools at your disposal!

Q. Are there any other benefits to the digestive tract with chitosan use?

A. Dr. Ward Dean, a physician in Florida, highly recommends that his patients suffering from inflammatory bowel disease take 1,500 mg of chitosan per meal to reduce their symptoms. His patients have found that the protective, healing qualities of chitosan help to reduce the amount of pain medication needed to control the pain caused by Crohn's disease or by ulcers. Dr. Dean speculates that chitosan is not only healing to the lining of the intestinal tract, but the added fiber gently keeps the intestinal tract clean and aids in the healing process of inflamed tissue.

Q. Can chitosan prevent any foreign materials from entering the body through the intestinal wall?

A. Chitosan may prevent certain bacteria and microorganisms from being absorbed through the intestinal wall, possibly because of its powerful positive-charge magnetics. Think of chitosan as a microorganism magnet that attracts a pathogenic, or disease-causing, organism to its surface, then escorts it out of the body. Chitosan is a kind of "bacteria bouncer"!

Because chitosan is a fiber, it moves through the intestinal tract, picking up other debris, and removes it from the body in the feces. This debris could include other types of residue on the foods that you would not want to be absorbed into the blood stream. But remember, for maximum effectiveness, you should not rely solely on chitosan as your dietary fiber. You should consume several forms of fiber to help perform this sweeping of your intestines.

Q. Does chitosan influence the immune system?

A. Unless you have an allergy to shellfish, in which case you should not use chitosan, it seems that chitosan's effects on the immune system are positive. Chitosan appears to play a role in helping activate IgM, one of the immunoglobulins produced by a healthy immune system in response to an attack by harmful bacteria or other invaders. High levels of the immunoglobulin indicates a current immune system challenge. Tests conducted *in vitro* showed that chitosan produced a strong IgM response, which could be helpful in supporting the immune system. However, it showed no influence on IgG or IgA antibodies.

4.

Incorporating Chitosan Into a Healthy Diet

A healthy weight-loss program will encourage you to examine your diet and help you make better menu choices from day to day. It will maximize your intake of the five macronutrients—carbohydrates, proteins, fats, water, and fiber—and your intake of all the essential micronutrients—vitamins, minerals, and enzymes. However, regardless of how committed you are to making good food selections, from time to time you may want to enjoy some fattening goodies—guilt-free! Incorporating chitosan into a healthy weight-loss plan can help you to "have your cake and eat it too"!

Q. What is considered a realistic weight-loss goal?

A. Optimally, you want to lose about one-half to one pound of fat weight per week. If you lose weight more rapidly, it is likely you will lose muscle tissue, particularly if you are not eating enough protein to maintain your lean muscle mass. However, if you eat a high-carbohydrate diet and increase the protein content up to optimum levels, you may lose ten to fifteen pounds of excess water weight within one to two weeks. A diet that is excessive in carbohydrates often leads to water retention, and when you reduce the carbohydrates and increase the protein, you may enjoy a brief period of losing excess water.

This weight loss should slow to about one-half to one pound of weight loss per week after the initial loss of ten to fifteen pounds.

Q. What should I eat while I'm using chitosan?

A. There is a great deal of controversy about

what constitutes a healthy diet. With all the conflicting information on nutrition being published, chances are you are very confused. Even government documents show some inconsistencies in how the food pyramid should be constructed. If the experts don't agree, how can the average American figure it out?

If you can put all the current diet theory aside and consider some nutrition facts, you will see that it is not difficult to put together a well-balanced meal program that will help you to lose weight. There are a few principles of nutrition that, once understood, will end your diet confusion forever.

One of these principles is that you must consume an adequate amount of protein each day to supply the basic building blocks for muscle and for the 300,000 different protein structures in your body. Another principle is that you should consume an adequate amount of carbohydrates each day to supply your body with enough energy to perform its functions. The other principles include consuming an adequate supply of essential fats, drinking a lot of water, taking in an adequate supply of fiber, and getting the required amounts of vitamins and minerals each day. Read on to discover how to do this.

Q. How much protein should I get from my diet?

A. Protein can be found in all animal foods and also in legumes, grains, and vegetables. The average woman needs between 45 and 75 g of protein each day, and the average man needs between 65 and 85 g of protein each day. Servings of protein foods should be divided between three meals per day, with a significant amount of protein served with breakfast.

I recommend that you purchase a high-quality protein supplement drink from your local health-food store to use as your breakfast drink. Most protein drinks are made from either a soy or a rice/vegetable source. These drinks should be low in sugars and should not contain any artificial ingredients, such as flavorings, sweeteners, or coloring agents. Use one tablespoon of flaxseed oil with your protein drink to supply the proper amount of essential fatty acids.

The average serving of animal protein contains about 9 g of protein per ounce, so if you require 45 g of protein daily, you will need about 5 ounces of animal protein each day, in divided doses. If you choose vegetarian sources of protein, it is particularly important that you work with a knowledgeable nutritionist who can help you combine vegetarian sources of protein to ensure that you receive adequate amounts of all the essential amino acids, vitamins, and minerals that are typically under-supplied in a vegetarian diet. You will also want to make sure you do not overconsume protein sources that are potential allergens, such as soy, eggs, and dairy.

Q. Are there any other considerations when choosing protein foods?

A. Proteins are comprised of individual amino acids, which are strung together to form very complex proteins. Protein, as it is eaten, is unusable to the body and must be broken down through digestion into the individual amino acids. There are about ten essential amino acids—essential means that your body does not produce them so you must get them in your diet. Each of the amino acids has a specific, unique role to play in the body; and it is critical that you eat adequate amounts of total protein and that all ten essential amino acids are well supplied. Animal proteins already contain an optimum balance of amino acids, so if you are consuming fish, chicken, or turkey, for example, you do not need to worry about essential amino acids. If, however, you have chosen a vegetarian lifestyle, you will need to carefully assess the amino acid composition of your diet to make sure you are receiving each one, in optimum amounts. It is helpful to work with a knowledgeable nutritionist to determine the best course of action for you.

Q. What about carbohydrates?

A. Another general principle regarding a healthy diet is that your body needs carbohydrates. Carbohydrates are just as important as protein, but the average American diet is oversupplied with refined, sugary carbohydrates. Average Americans also eat too many refined grain products, such as bagels, pasta, bread, and cereal. The reason most people gain unwanted weight is that they overdo the carbohydrates. For the most part, carbohydrates make you gain weight!

Carbohydrates supply the brain and the rest of the body with energy, so it is essential that you consume enough carbohydrates to fuel your active brain and body. To help you choose good sources of carbohydrates, let me offer some simple rules:

First, eliminate all processed grains from your diet. In fact, while you are trying to lose weight, eliminate *all* grains from your diet! This will reduce your carbohydrate intake and reduce the intake of potential allergens that may be causing you to gain weight.

Second, enjoy a wide variety of vegetables with your lunch and evening meals. Enjoy a salad tossed with olive oil and balsamic vinegar, for example. If you eat potatoes or carrots, only include a tiny portion of these starchy foods and make up the difference in brightly colored vegetables, such as broccoli, peppers, jicama, green beans, and onions. Plan to eat at least five servings of fresh vegetables each day. Your body will love you for it! Vegetables provide your brain and your body with the energy and the micronutrients needed for vibrant, sparkling health!

Q. Do I need to reduce my fat intake to have a healthy diet?

A. This seems like such a simple question, but

the issue of dietary fats is much more complex than simply removing them from your diet. It is difficult to understand how very essential fat is by reading popular literature! You may be surprised to know that fat is actually an essential part of the diet and that the body uses it for hundreds of structures and functions in the body. For example, it is the preferred source of energy for the heart; it is used to produce hundreds of hormones and neurotransmitters; it maintains a healthy hormone level; it aids in the transmission of nerve messages; it is used to maintain a healthy cell wall membrane to allow entry of nutrients into the cell and to escort toxic materials out of the cell; and it has hundreds of other functions. Studies show that Americans are actually deficient in many types of essential fats and oils. One of the side effects of inadequate amounts of essential fatty acids is lowered metabolism—resulting in weight gain!

Q. Now I'm really confused! Shouldn't getting rid of fat be the solution to my weight problem?

A. Getting rid of the highly processed, free-radical-producing rancid fats is a major part of the solution. But consuming proper amounts of natural, minimally processed raw oil is extremely beneficial and will actually help you to lose weight.

Eating 1 to 2 tablespoons of high-quality oil each day in the form of olive oil, flaxseed oil, butter, or the fats found in raw nuts and seeds, avocados, deep-sea fish, and some other foods is very important to a healthy diet. However, you will want to be sure to eliminate all sources of toxic oils, or oils that have been highly processed, heated to high temperatures, or chemically altered in other ways. Some of the most damaging oils are those found in vegetable oils or salad oils, margarine or other hydrogenated fat products, bacon or other aged meats, pseudo-cheese products, and homogenized dairy products.

Q. What about my vitamin and mineral intake?

A. If you have dieted frequently over the past few months or years, it is likely that you are suffering from micronutrient deficiencies that will sabotage your efforts to lose weight. Make sure that you use a high-quality vitamin supplement and mineral supplement that will make up for past and current deficiencies. It is especially important that the supplement contain triple-digit amounts of calcium, magnesium, and chromium—for example, 400 mcg of chromium or 500 mg of calcium, and double-digit amounts of zinc and other trace minerals—15 mg of zinc, for example.

Q. How much water should I drink?

A. When you use a fiber supplement such as chitosan, it is doubly important that you drink at least eight to ten 8-ounce glasses of pure water each day. Divide your water goal into eight even parts and space it throughout the day so you are hydrating your entire body, not just running it through your kidneys by drinking it all at one time. Drink a little extra water with your chitosan supplement to make sure that it remains soft as it passes through your body.

Q. How much fiber do I need?

A. Nutritionists recommend that you consume

about 30 g of fiber each day. The average American consumes only about 5 to 6 g of fiber per day—far too little to maintain a healthy colon and lower blood fats. You can get an adequate amount of fiber from your food if you eat at least five servings of fresh vegetables each day. Beans are an especially rich source of fiber.

Unfortunately, most of us don't eat enough vegetables to supply the required amounts of fiber, so it becomes necessary to supplement our fiber intake. Chitosan will serve well as additional fiber. You may also wish to use a powdered fiber that does not contain added sugars, which is available at your local health-food store. If it contains acidophilus and other friendly bacteria, so much the better. This powdered fiber can be mixed with the protein breakfast drink in the morning for a smooth texture and a rich supply of beneficial fiber.

Q. Can you summarize all that diet information for me?

A. Include an adequate amount of the following macronutrients in your diet: protein (45 to 65 g for women and 65 to 85 g for men); carbohydrates (5 to 7 servings of fresh vegetables per day); fats (1 to 2 tablespoons of raw, unprocessed oils each day); water (eight to ten 8-ounce glasses per day); fiber (up to 30 g per day); vitamin and minerals (choose a well-balanced supplement that contains all essential nutrients in significant amounts).

Q. How does chitosan fit into a healthy well-balanced diet that promotes weight loss?

A. As we have learned, chitosan reduces the absorption of fats so that they are escorted out of the body before they can be stored as body fat. Chitosan works well as a supplement to a healthy diet by reducing the amount of harmful fats that are absorbed and stored by the body and also by reducing the amount of calories from these fats.

We have seen how important essential fatty acids are, and that many people do not get enough of these essential fatty acids in their diets. It is, therefore, important that when you use chitosan, you only use it before eating a meal that is loaded with processed, rancid fats, and not with a meal that is rich in the essential fatty acids. For example, if you have chosen to use the protein breakfast drink and decide to use flaxseed oil in the drink to provide a portion of essential oils, do *not* use the chitosan at the same time. However, if you've chosen a breakfast consisting of bacon and eggs, French toast soaked in butter, a bagel with cream cheese, or a ham and cheese omelet with fried hash browns, you may wish to use chitosan at the beginning of the meal to absorb the harmful fats you will be consuming.

An additional example of this advice would be if you have chosen a brightly colored salad with dark green lettuce, peppers, onions, and shredded carrots with an Italian dressing (made from extra virgin olive oil) and tuna packed in water, you will not want to use the chitosan because it would absorb the healthy oils found in those foods. If, however, you've chosen to lunch at your local greasy spoon or your neighborhood fast-food restaurant—even the salad dressings at fast-food restaurants are loaded with highly processed, unhealthy fats—you may wish to use the chitosan before the meal to absorb the rancid fats that are found in that meal selection.

So you see, you will need to think carefully about your meal selections, and tailor your use of chitosan to your dietary choices.

Q. Will eating a rich dessert occasionally spoil my healthy diet?

A. Again, this is where chitosan can be of value to the conscientious eater. No one eats a perfectly healthy diet all the time. Even the most dedicated nutritionist likes to indulge occasionally in something he or she may consider forbidden. When you are on your weight-loss regimen, you will find it helpful if you regulate your intake of these forbidden foods. In other words, you don't swear off everything totally, forever. You may decide that once per week, you can satisfy your sweet tooth with a fat-rich brownie or a bowl of ice cream, or you can be contented with a Saturday night bowl of buttery popcorn. Choose one night per week as your "treat night"—and enjoy yourself without feeling guilty. To reduce the fat that will be absorbed by your body from this treat, use chitosan just before dipping into that bowl of popcorn or that dish of ice cream— a substantial portion of the fat will be escorted out of the body before it can do damage to your waistline!

Remember that dietary rigidity is doomed to dietary failure. A little flexibility will psychologically and physically help you to cope with the rigors of changing your eating habits. Chitosan may help to make that transition a little easier for you!

Chitosan is not meant to be used as a substitute for good eating habits. It is like any other dietary supplement—a support tool or a crutch to help you through the difficult times. And in that sense, chitosan is not the "magic pill" that will make all the fat go away. It is there to support you as you are learning to eat properly and as you are learning how to balance your calorie intake with your calorie use.

Q. How much chitosan should I take?

A. To help you lower the amount of fat taken into the body, Dr. Ivan Furda recommends you use 3 to 4 g of chitosan each day, in divided doses. In other words, you would take about 1 g of chitosan per meal, assuming that particular meal contains harmful fats that need to be removed. This dosage of 3 to 4 g of chitosan will remove up to 10 to 15 g of fat daily, resulting in a net loss of up to 500 calories! Or better yet, use chitosan only when you choose to indulge in a high-fat meal. No research has been published on the long-term effects of using a fiber supplement to remove large amounts of fat from the diet, so prudence indicates that you do not use chitosan on a daily basis.

Q. How can I be sure that I'm purchasing a good quality chitosan product?

A. Currently, there are no specific standards for chitosan manufacturing or in the labeling of chitosan products. It is clear that there are many forms of both chitin and chitosan and that some forms work better for some uses than others.

In addition to its supplemental form, chitosan is also available for external applications. These applications will be discussed in Chapter 6. Whatever form you choose, it is important that you purchase chitosan from a manufacturer who uses good manufacturing practices (GMP). Your supplement provider or cosmetic company should be able to supply you with this information.

5.

The Pros and Cons
of Chitosan Use

You've read about the incredible benefits that chitosan can bring to the frustrated dieter by reducing the amount of fat absorbed, so that calories can be lowered and weight loss can result. You've also read about chitosan's additional qualities, such as the ability to lower cholesterol and triglycerides, to reduce the risk of certain types of cancer, to normalize blood sugar in diabetics, and to increase the response of the immune system. However, like any natural product, there are a few cautions to be taken. Even natural, beneficial substances can be misused or overused, so it is important to understand both the pros and cons of using a powerful substance like chitosan.

Q. Is chitosan considered to be a safe product?

A. An article published in the *Journal of Biomedical Materials Research* states that chitosan is safe. Human toxicity tests were conducted to determine chitosan's safety, and the report reads, "In vivo toxicity tests indicated that it is nontoxic." However, with any product, whether it's natural or not, adverse reactions may occur because of allergies and sometimes because of unknown reasons. If you are allergic to shellfish, for example, you must use extreme caution and must get your doctor's permission before using chitosan. The standard recommendation for trying any new product is to start slowly, increase your intake slowly, and pay close attention to your body's reaction.

Q. Who can potentially benefit from the use of chitosan?

A. The people who will benefit most from chitosan use are individuals who are committed to pursuing a healthy diet but need to lose a significant amount of weight. They have tried calorie- or fat-reducing diets in the past and have been frustrated by their seemingly insatiable appetite for fatty foods. They are not looking for an excuse for sloppy, self-indulgent eating habits, but simply need a little help while they are getting their eating habits under control. These are the people who are overweight because they really do eat too many calories in the form of rancid, highly processed fats and oil.

Q. What types of weight problems can't be helped by taking chitosan?

A. If you are considering using chitosan to help you lose weight, you may wish to learn more about why you are struggling with weight and honestly assess your own situation. For example, if you are female and your weight is primarily centered between your waist and your knees and you are relatively thin above the waist and below the knees, you are probably overweight as a result of excess estrogen—you may be perimenopausal or postmenopausal; you may be using estrogen replacement therapy or birth control pills; or you may be suffering from a hormone imbalance from another origin. If you are going to successfully lose weight, chitosan will probably not help you. In this case, you will need to ask your nutritionally oriented physician for his or her recommendations for balancing your hormones.

If you are male and your body has an apple shape because of excess weight—for example, your weight is primarily above your abdomen and around your chest—you probably eat too many carbohydrates and may benefit from following the diet recommendations in the previous chapter. (Chitosan may help you drop a few pounds, as well.)

If you are struggling with an underactive thyroid, chitosan supplementation may make your symptoms worse if you lower your fat intake too dramatically. It may also reduce your metabolic rate even further.

If your weight problem is caused by your body's response to allergens in your diet—primarily wheat and dairy products—you will need to eliminate those products from your diet to successfully lose weight.

Q. Can children use chitosan?

A. Children should not use chitosan because an adequate amount of dietary fat is essential for the development of their nervous systems, their brains, and their hormone systems. It is important to teach children to reduce the amount of harmful fats in the diet and to enjoy beneficial fats, rather than to teach them to artificially manipulate the fats in their diets. Using chitosan may send a harmful message to children—that there is a "pill for every ill" and that selecting healthy foods is not important. Children should not be led to believe that they can solve the problem of poor food choices without exercising restraint and wisdom. They should be taught to understand that they can be thin and healthy by eating correctly— and they will enjoy the benefits of these choices for the rest of their lives!

Q. Can pregnant or lactating women use chitosan?

A. Pregnant and lactating women should not use chitosan because a balance of good fats and oils is critical to development of a baby's brain and nervous system. Studies have shown that deficiencies in omega-3 fatty acids, for example, can lead to permanent damage to a baby's brain. In addition, pregnant and lactating women need a high-energy diet to keep them healthy and strong during pregnancy and breastfeeding. These periods require a lot of energy, so there is a need for the extra calories acquired from beneficial oils and a high-calorie diet.

The periods during pregnancy and breastfeeding are not the time for a new mom to go on a diet!

Q. Is there anyone else who should not use chitosan?

A. Anyone who has an allergy to shellfish should not use chitosan because it is taken from the shells of crabs, shrimp, and other crustaceans. Those who are suffering from an extreme allergy must be especially careful to avoid all forms of chitosan to eliminate the possibility of triggering an allergic reaction. While the proteins in the chitosan have been removed and proteins are what usually trigger allergic reactions, you should still avoid chitosan if you are allergic to shellfish.

Q. What about people with low cholesterol levels?

A. Most people do not realize that low levels of cholesterol are just as dangerous as high levels of cholesterol. Studies show that people whose cholesterol levels are too low—under 130 mg/dl, for example—are at a higher risk of developing certain forms of cancer, or are more prone to depression or episodes of violent behavior.

Although some media have promoted the concept of "the lower the better" regarding blood cholesterol levels, the fact is that cholesterol levels should range from 170 mg/dl to 220 mg/dl. Please see your doctor for his or her advice about your personal cholesterol levels.

Q. If chitosan prevents my body from absorbing harmful fats, will it also prevent my body from absorbing essential fats and other nutrients?

A. Chitosan is non-selective in the removal of fats. In other words, in the presence of chitosan, all fats are at risk for being escorted out of the intestinal tract, even the essential fatty acids. Fat-soluble vitamins, such as vitamins A, D, E, and K, are also at risk for being escorted out of your system. Other minerals—such as calcium, which absorbs better in the presence of fat and vitamin D—are dependent upon fat in the diet for absorption. This is why it is important not to take chitosan with every meal and why you must take an active role in your weight-loss program.

In Chapter 4, you learned the importance of balancing your diet with the adequate amounts of protein, carbohydrates, water, fiber, *and* essential fats. The most important concept to understand in the controversy over dietary fat is that not all fats are nutritionally equal. You should take chitosan before meals that contain harmful fats, such as those found in fast food, snack food, salad dressing, desserts, and nearly every processed food. You should not take chitosan before meals that contain essential fats, such as those found in olive oil, flaxseed oil, avocados, raw nuts and seeds, deep-sea fish, and other natural foods.

Q. What do studies show about chitosan and nutrient removal?

A. The Kirin Brewery Company in Japan performed a study on rats to assess the effect of high and continuous intake of chitosan on mineral and vitamin status and found that chitosan "led to a marked and rapid decrease in the serum vitamin E level." This study also reported that "Chitosan feeding for two weeks caused a decrease in mineral absorption and bone mineral content, and it was necessary to administer twice the amount of Ca (calcium) . . . to prevent such a decrease in the bone mineral content."

While the chitosan content of the rats' diet was especially high—probably higher than most humans would consume by choice—it should be noted that you may run the risk of depleting valuable vitamin and mineral status by "continuous and high" intake of chitosan. If you are going to use chitosan, therefore, plan to use it just for meals that are high in harmful fats. You should not use chitosan at every meal. Be selective in your use!

Q. How can I avoid decreased absorption of my vitamin and mineral supplements while I'm using chitosan?

A. It is critically important that you take your vitamin and mineral supplements—including flaxseed oil and other essential fatty acids—at a meal in which you are not using chitosan. Plan to space your chitosan intake and your supplement intake at least six hours apart to give your body the chance to absorb the nutrients. For example, you may choose to take your vitamin and mineral supplements with your protein breakfast drink mixed with flaxseed oil, then take chitosan before your high-fat evening meal to help ensure an optimum essential nutrient status in your body.

Several studies indicate that the use of chitosan itself increased the body's requirement for minerals and other nutrients. Therefore, during the period of time that you are using chitosan, it would be prudent for you to take higher amounts of your supplements to compensate for possible loss of nutrients in the fiber mix.

Q. Are there any other contraindications for using chitosan?

A. If you have been a frequent dieter, you need to be careful not to lower your calorie intake too quickly, otherwise you could jeopardize your body's ability to burn fat as energy. We know that lowering the fat allowance in the diet too drastically reduces the metabolic rate of the body—the speed at which your body burns calories. Over the long haul, this will, of course, make it increasingly difficult to lose weight and keep it off. So, if your goal is permanent weight loss, it is vitally important that you follow the diet recommendations in Chapter 4, especially if you choose to supplement your diet with chitosan.

There is no value in continuing to lower calorie content below that which your body requires to maintain its internal energy. There is no virtue in starvation.

Q. Do any nutrients help chitosan become even more effective in fat removal?

A. It seems that using vitamin C along with chitosan may actually lead to increased inhibition of fat digestion and absorption. A study published in *Bioscience, Biotechnology, and Biochemistry* investigated the mechanism for the inhibition of fat digestion and the synergistic effect of ascorbate, or vitamin C. Researchers believe that there are several reasons for this synergistic effect, one of which is that vitamin C seems to make the clump of chitosan and fat more flexible and less likely to leak entrapped fat into the intestinal tract.

The type of vitamin C used in the study was sodium ascorbate, a form of vitamin C that can be obtained from your health-food store.

6.

Other Health-Related Uses of Chitosan

In addition to being a dietary supplement, chitosan has been used for diverse purposes, such as purifying waste water, cleaning up oil-slicks, and readying cotton fibers for dyeing. But more recently, researchers have been studying how chitosan can play a valuable role in human health unrelated to dietary intake. They have found that because of its unique properties, Chitosan can be used in topical applications and also in drug delivery systems.

Q. In what way is chitosan used for topical applications?

A. Because chitosan has several unique bio-chemical properties, it is well suited in cosmetic use and hair treatments. As mentioned previously, chitosan is a positively charged molecule at a pH of about 6, which means that it is slightly acidic. When it retains its positive charge, the tissue is very similar to that of skin and hair, making it an ideal feature in hair products. For example, chitosan tends to form films with the hair's natural keratins, making its coating action more stable at high humidity. Chitosan-treated hair shows less tendency to stick together, and because it is not as electrically charged, it is easier to brush and keep in place. In addition, the clear protective coating of chitosan protects hair strength and helps hair maintain its luster.

Q. Can chitosan be used on my skin as well?

A. Because chitosan can hold both water and oil, it is perfect for topical use on the skin and in skin-care products, such as acne creams, lotions, emollients, and suntan lotions. Chitosan forms a protective film to protect the skin from environmental assaults and helps retain both oil and water moisture in the skin. Chitosan has roughly the same pH of the skin—slightly acidic—helping the skin maintain its normal pH balance, which is essential for skin health. When chitosan is applied in a thin layer, it gently adheres to the area, protecting it. In fact, it actually readily binds to the skin, making it suitable for a variety of biomedical and cosmetic uses.

Q. Can bacteria get under the protective layer of chitosan and cause infection?

A. Chitosan has been shown to be bacteriostatic—it kills bacteria and other types of microorganisms on contact. This substance is also known to be hemostatic, meaning that it reduces the flow of the blood. It could, therefore, be used to stop the flow of blood in a minor injury and protect it from becoming infected.

Q. Can chitosan be used as a burn treatment?

A. Because of its ability to form a fairly tough, water-absorbent film over the surface of the skin, scientists are currently investigating the use of chitosan for the treatment of burns. First, the chitosan is dissolved in water, then it is applied to the surface of the skin in a thin layer. Even though the mixture is slightly acidic, it feels cool to the open wounds of burn victims. Oxygen is allowed to penetrate through the chitosan, allowing for faster healing.

Furthermore, after the wound is healed, the chitosan does not need to be removed because the enzymes in the skin naturally break down this substance. As a result, the delicate healing tissues are not damaged by the removal of a bandage.

Q. How is a wound treated with chitosan?

A. Dr. Ward Dean, who practices in Florida, counsels his patients suffering from a second-degree burn—where there is blistering and weeping of the damaged skin tissue—to open a capsule of chitosan and gently sprinkle the powder over the wound, completely covering it. The antibacterial properties of the chitosan reduce the possibility of a bacterial infection and keep the area clean while it heals. Eventually, the chitosan is broken down and absorbed by the body, making removal from the tender area unnecessary.

Q. Can chitosan be used for internal wound healing, as well?

A. Scientists are considering using chitosan to help build prosthetic structures—replacements for bone, cartilage, arteries, veins, and musculo-fascial replacements. Because chitin is compatible with living skin and has the ability to form sulfate esters that reduce the risk of blood clot formation, it may potentially be used for helping to sculpture replacement tissue. As one researcher put it, "The uses of chitin and chitosan are only limited by the creativity of the biomedical engineer."

Q. Have pharmaceutical companies looked at some possible applications for chitosan?

A. A number of studies have been conducted using chitosan as a vehicle for the delivery of certain forms of drugs into the body. One of the challenges that pharmaceutical researchers face is how to get a specific drug to a specific site in the body without losing its effectiveness in the digestive tract or the liver, and without damaging other organs in the process.

One study conducted in India tested a cancer drug using chitosan as a type of carrier molecule. Mitoxantrone, an antineoplastic agent, was inserted into chitosan microspheres and injected into mice to test how well it worked against a specific type of cancerous tumor—Ehrlich ascites carcinoma. The mean survival time of the mice that were treated with the free mitoxantrone—without the use of chitosan—was between two and five days. The mean survival time of the mice treated with the injections of chitosan microspheres was fifty days—five out of eight lived beyond sixty days. Researchers also noted that drug toxicity was minimized while achieving maximum therapeutic efficacy.

Q. Will chitosan work as a delivery system for other forms of drugs?

A. A number of drugs have been studied in connection with chitosan as a delivery system. For example, researchers in Saudi Arabia filled chitosan microspheres with phenobarbitone—otherwise known as phenobarbital—a drug used as a sedative, a hypnotic, and an anticonvulsant. Though phenobarbital is usually administered orally, researchers wanted to see if the microsphere would alter the rate of delivery of this powerful drug into the body. They found that there was an initial rapid release of the drug, 20 to 30 percent, then the remaining portion of the drug was released slowly. Time-releasing a powerful drug of this nature can ease some of the side effects that accompany its usage, thereby making it more effective.

An example of this time-release effect can be seen in the work done in Italy at the Universita di Pavia. In this study, ampicillin—a form of antibiotic—was embedded in microparticles made from a new derivative of chitosan called methylpyrrolidinone chitosan. The drug-loaded particles were then spray-dried and laboratory tested against different types of bacteria. Again, researchers found that the drug was released over a period of time and either maintained or improved the antibacterial activity of the drug.

One additional study done in India used the steroids testosterone, progesterone, and estrogen mixed with chitosan, then dried. While these tests were not done on humans to determine how rapidly the drug was released, it showed that the microbeads stayed intact for a longer period of time in dissolution tests, and the possibility of using this type of delivery system for contraceptive purposes was discussed.

Q. Can chitosan microspheres help to prevent drugs from being prematurely released into the body?

A. Researchers at the University of Santiago de Compostela in Spain used chitosan as a microencapsulation microsphere to test if drugs could be safely escorted all the way to the colon without digesting in the stomach or small intestine. This test was quite complicated due to the varying degrees of acidity in different sections of the digestive tract. Researchers used sodium diclofenac as a model drug and encased it in microspheres of chitosan, which were then further encased in other materials that would not be degraded in the acid environment of the stomach. After successfully moving through the stomach, the spheres reached the colon, where the bacteria in the colon broke them down, releasing the drug into the alkaline environment of the colon. This was the result that researchers were expecting.

Q. Does chitosan have any other uses in the preparation of drugs?

A. Because chitosan is biodegradable and biocompatible, it can be effectively used in the preparation of tablets or capsules as a pharmaceutical excipient. An excipient is an inert substance that has been added to a tablet or capsule to help achieve a suitable consistency and to make the tablet more palatable to the user.

Pharmaceutical companies in the United Kingdom and Japan are using chitosan to help compress tablets, to help tablets disintegrate, and to prepare controlled released drugs. Researchers noted that "Chitosan has, compared to traditional excipients, been shown to have superior characteristics and especially flexibility in its use." They are exploring other uses for this "exciting and promising excipient" in the future, including for the delivery of hormones.

Q. Do you have any anecdotes about chitosan use?

A. Mark Ludlow of Natural Biopolymer Inc.,

told the story of a cat who had an unfortunate encounter with a car and suffered massive wounds. The cat was scheduled to be euthanized, but its loving owners looked for a better solution. The wound area where the flesh was missing was packed with chitosan fibers, cleaned, and bandaged. Apparently, the chitosan acted as a type of template for the growth of new cell formation. Within twenty-three days, the cat's wounds had healed, without a scar. Certainly, that was good news for the cat and its owner, but it could be good news for all of us!

It is likely that as chitosan research continues to be conducted, new and potentially exciting uses will be found for this extremely abundant, flexible material.

7.

Agricultural and Industrial Uses of Chitosan

In the 1970s, interest in natural fibers took the spotlight, and research began on the use of chitosan in water purification plants and in other non-dietary applications, such as biomedical applications, paper production, agriculture, textile finishes, photographic products, cements, heavy metal chelating agents, and waste removal. Time and time again, chitosan has proven to be a truly versatile fiber!

Q. How is chitosan used in water purification plants?

A. Scientists have found that treating water that

has been contaminated with heavy metals or oil—as in accidents involving oil-carrying tankers, for example—is expensive, time consuming, and not very effective. So researchers at the Massachusetts Institute of Technology (MIT) are pioneering the use of chitosan in removing these harmful materials from both ground water and bodies of water that have been polluted. In a process called chemically enhanced primary treatment (CEPT), small amounts of chemicals are added to raw sewage, which causes the particulate matter in the sewage to clump together and fall to the bottom of the water. Researchers have found that the magnetic force of chitosan can hold the metals "captive," and thus substitute for the chemicals normally used in this primary treatment plan. Because chitosan sells for about seven dollars per pound, it reduces cost, and is a more effective means of water treatment.

Q. How is chitosan used in textile preparation?

A. Cotton is the most commonly used natural textile fiber in the world, accounting for about 50 percent of the total world fiber production. High-quality cotton is used for apparel use, while the lower quality cotton is sent to industrial applications.

Cotton growers in the Southern High Plains of Texas produce about 52 percent of the state's cotton, which is used by textile mills throughout the world. The problem with cotton grown in this region is that it contains a high percentage of small knots or fiber entanglements called neps, which prevent the cotton from adequately absorbing dyes, thus increasing the cost of production and lowering the amount of cotton available to the clothing industry.

The industry has found that pretreating cotton fibers with chitosan allows the dye to be received by the fibers more uniformly. This pretreatment plan still tends to be costly because the industry must pretreat all cotton fabrics before dyeing. Using chitosan in an after-treatment, however, was found to be cost effective, especially for fabrics already rejected because of the presence of neps.

Chitin has also been studied as a possible way to remove dyes and metal ions from textile effluent or waste materials.

Q. What other industrial and agricultural uses does chitosan have?

A. Researchers are looking into the possibility of using chitosan in place of oil emulsions for the controlled release of pesticides, biofertilizers, and biochemicals into soil.

In agriculture, it is possible that chitosan can also be used as a protective agent for plants, for seed coating, and for fruit preservation. When chitin is used in potato farming, the result is a product that is less watery, and thus, better tasting.

Conclusion

Nearly every day we hear another message about how important it is to cut the fat out of our diets, to lower our calorie intake, and to bring our diets into compliance with the recommendations made by consensus of nutritionists and doctors. Even the federal government gets involved by trying to raise the standard of the American diet. But following right behind this barrage of words about why it is important to clean up our diets is another set of messages from television and other popular media that entices us to buy another tasty treat. The voice in one ear shouts, "Shape up! Get your diet under control!" while the voice in the other ear yells, "C'mon! You can eat just one!" Stuck in the middle is the hapless consumer who is driven by his own internal hunger to eat what shouldn't be eaten. The consumer cries, "I don't want to give up my favorite food, even if it is bad for me!"

Chitosan promises to become the bridge between these two drives, a type of crutch to help us reduce the absorption of fat from highly processed fatty foods while we relearn our eating habits. Trying to unlearn a deeply ingrained habit is not easy. It isn't done overnight, and it isn't done just by gritting our teeth and fighting our way through it. It is more easily accomplished by relying on a natural product that can help by letting a little of those harmful fats slip through the body unnoticed.

Chitosan isn't a magic bullet. It isn't the pill that makes all the dietary ills go away, and it certainly isn't an excuse for unhealthy food choices. But when used responsibly, chitosan can be a dieter's true friend. Undeniably, the secret to permanent, healthy weight loss is a lifelong commitment to healthy eating habits. However, when those urgent cravings for something rich and fatty scream for satisfaction, chitosan is available to escort the excess fat out of the body and out of harm's way.

Glossary

Cation. An ion carrying a positive electrical charge.

Cellulose. The principal component of wood; a type of polysaccharide that is indigestible in the human body.

Chitin. One of the most abundant natural biopolymers in the world, second only to cellulose. It is a naturally occurring polysaccharide that contains amino sugars, and is found in crustacean shells, insect exoskeletons, fungal cell walls, microfauna, and plankton.

Chitosan. The deacetylated derivative of chitin. Chitosan has been used extensively in research. The deacetylation renders chitosan more useful in applications.

Essential fatty acids. Fats, or lipids, that cannot be manufactured by the body, but must be supplied in the diet, and play both structural and functional roles in the body.

Polymer. A compound formed by combining smaller molecules, such as polypeptides, polysaccharides, and nucleic acids.

Polysaccharide. A carbohydrate consisting of a large number of saccharide groups. Cellulose and chitin are polysaccharides. Polysaccharides are distributed abundantly throughout the food chain as fibers, and are, for the most part, indigestible.

References

Deuchi K, Kanauchi O, Shizukuishi M, Kobayashi E, "Continuous and massive intake of chitosan affects mineral and fat-soluble vitamin status in rats fed on a high-fat diet," *Bioscience, Biotechnology, and Biochemistry* 59(7)(July 1995):1211–1216.

Ebihara K, Schneeman BO, "Interaction of bile acids, phospholipids, cholesterol and triglycerides with dietary fibers in the small intestine of rats," *Journal of Nutrition* 119(8)(Aug 1989):1100–1106.

Furda, Ivan, PhD, "Aminopolysaccharides—Their Potential as Dietary Fiber," *American Chemical Society*, 1983.

Ikeda I, Tomari Y, Sugano M, "Interrelated effects of dietary fiber and fat on lymphatic cholesterol and triglyceride absorption in rats," *Journal of Nutrition* 119(10)(Oct 1989):1383–1387.

Kanauchi O, Deuchi K, Imasato Y, Shizukuishi M, Kobayashi E, "Mechanism for the inhibition of fat digestion by chitosan and for the synergistic effect of ascorbate," *Bioscience, Biotechnology, and Biochemistry* 59(5)(May 1995):786–790.

Landes DR, Bough WA, "Effects of chitosan—a coagulating agent for food processing wastes—in the diets of rats on growth and liver and blood composition," *Bulletin of Environmental Contaminants and Toxicology* 1(5)(May 1976):555–563.

LeHoux JG, Grondin F, "Some effects of chitosan on liver function in the rat," *Endocrinology* 132(3) (March 1993):1078–1084.

Lorenzo-Lamosa ML, Remunan-Lopez C, Vila-Jato JL, Alonso MJ, "Design of microencapsulated chitosan microspheres for colonic drug delivery," *Journal of Controlled Release* 52(1–2)(March 1998):109–118.

Maeda M, Murakami H, Ohta H, Tajima M, "Stimulation of IgM production in human-human hybridoma HB4C5 cells by chitosan," *Bioscience, Biotechnology, and Biochemistry* 56(3)(March 1992): 427–431.

Miura T, Usami M, Tsuura Y, Ishida H, Seino Y, "Hypoglycemic and hypolipidemic effect of chitosan in normal and neonatal streptozotocin-induced diabetic mice," *Biological Pharmaceutical Bulletin* 18(11)(November 1995):1623–1625.

Mueller Jennifer, "Chitosan—A Brief Overview," *Vitamin Research Product's Nutritional News*, July/August, 1995.

Okunevich IV, Kliueva NN, Solov'eva MA, Triufanov VF, Ryzhenkov VE, "The hypolipidemic effect of natural substances," *Eksp. Klin. Farmokol* 55(5)(September-October 1992):44–47.

Rao SB, Sharma CP, "Use of chitosan as a biomaterial: studies on its safety and hemostatic potential," *Journal of Biomedical Materials Research* (January 1997):21–28.

Razdan A, Pettersson D, "Effect of chitin and chitosan on nutrient digestibility and plasma lipid concentrations in broiler chickens," *British Journal Of Nutrition* 72(2)(August 1994):277–288.

Razdan A, Pettersson D, Pettersson J, "Broiler chicken body weight, feed intakes, plasma lipid and small-intestinal bile acid concentrations in response to feeding of chitosan and pectin," *British Journal of Nutrition* (August 1997):283-291.

Telephone interview with Marie Badde, PhD, November 2, 1998.

Telephone interview with Ward Dean, MD, November 2, 1998.

Telephone interview with Mark Ludlow, BS, November 5, 1998.

Torzsas TL, Kendall CW, Sugano M, Iwamoto Y, Rao AV, "The influence of high and low molecular weight chitosan on colonic cell proliferation and aberrant crypt foci development in CF1 mice," *Food Chemistry Toxicology* 34(1)(January 1996):73–77.

Vahouny GV, Satchithanandam S, Cassidy MM, Lightfoot FB, Furda I "Comparative effects of chitosan and cholestyramine on lymphatic absorption of lipids in the rat." *American Journal of Clinical Nutrition* 38(2)(August 1983):278–284.

Suggested Readings

Bellerson, Karen J. *The Complete and Up-to-Date Fat Book—3rd Edition.* Garden City Park, NY: Avery Publishing Group, 1997

Bellerson, Karen J. *The Shopper's Guide to Fat in Your Food.* Garden City Park, NY: Avery Publishing Group, 1994.

Rose, Gloria. *Low-Fat Cooking for Good Health.* Garden City Park, NY: Avery Publishing Group, 1996.

Simontacchi, Carol N., CCN, MS. *Your Fat Is Not Your Fault.* Los Angeles: Jeremy P. Tarcher/Putnam, 1998.

Woodruff, Sandra. *Secrets of Fat-Free Cooking.* Garden City Park, NY: Avery Publishing Group, 1998.

Woodruff, Sandra. *Secrets of Fat-Free Desserts.* Garden City Park, NY: Avery Publishing Group, 1998.

Index